AF885065

FAMILY MEDS ORGANIZER: A SIMPLE DAILY LOG FOR TRACKING MULTIPLE PRESCRIPTIONS

Stay on Schedule, Prevent Missed Doses, and Keep Everyone's Medication Information in One Place

By: DigiMedical

PUBLISHED BY: ADALYNN JAMES PUBLISHING
Blue Ash, OH 45242
www.adalynnjames.com

ADALYNN JAMES

Medication Hacks & Encouragement for Busy Families

Caring for your loved ones, especially when multiple family members are sick, can be overwhelming. Here are a few simple tips and words of encouragement to make the process easier and help you stay on track.

Smart Medication Hacks:

- □ Color-Code Medications: Use different colored stickers or labels for each child to prevent mix-ups.
- □ Use Alarms or Timers: Set phone reminders for each dose especially antibiotics that must stay on schedule.
- □ Designate a "Medication Station": Keep everything in one spot with measuring cups, syringes, paper towels, and water.
- □ Track Symptoms Daily: Write down any changes. This logbook has space to track this for each person.
- □ Double-check doses before giving, especially at night.
- □ Keep a backup thermometer and measuring tools handy.
- □ Use a pill organizer (label with times).
- □ Always finish the antibiotic unless the doctor told you to stop or there is an allergic reaction: Even if they feel better, stay strong and follow through!

Encouragement for You:

You're doing something powerful by keeping your family safe and organized. Whether you're a parent, caregiver, or guardian, your attention to detail helps prevent errors and gives your loved ones the care they need. You've got this—and we're proud of you.
Take it one day at a time. Keep logging, keep loving.

— DigiMedical, by Adalynn James Publishing

⚠ What to Do About Adverse Reactions ⚠

Sometimes medications cause unexpected side effects or allergic reactions. Knowing what to look for and what to do can save time and protect your loved ones.

Common Signs of a Reaction:

- Rash, hives, or swelling
- Difficulty breathing
- Vomiting or diarrhea
- Unusual sleepiness or irritability
- Dizziness or confusion

What to Do:

- Stop the medication immediately.
- Call your healthcare provider or local pharmacist for guidance.
- In case of emergency, dial 911 or go to the nearest Emergency Department.
- Record the reaction in this logbook to prevent future issues.

Notes about any reactions or questions to ask the doctor:

____

____

____

Name:
Allergies:

Date	Medication	Reaction

Name:
Allergies:

Date	Medication	Reaction

Name:
Allergies:

Date	Medication	Reaction

Name:
Allergies:

Date	Medication	Reaction

Name:
Allergies:

Date	Medication	Reaction

Name:
Allergies:

Date	Medication	Reaction

Name:
Allergies:

Date	Medication	Reaction

Name:
Allergies:

Date	Medication	Reaction

Name:

Doctor, Clinic, Hospital Contacts

Provider's Name	Contact Information

Doctor Appointment Log

Provider's Name	Speciality	Reason	Date/Time

Name:
Doctor, Clinic, Hospital Contacts

Provider's Name	Contact Information

Doctor Appointment Log

Provider's Name	Speciality	Reason	Date/Time

Name:
Doctor, Clinic, Hospital Contacts

Provider's Name	Contact Information

Doctor Appointment Log

Provider's Name	Speciality	Reason	Date/Time

Name:

Doctor, Clinic, Hospital Contacts

Provider's Name	Contact Information

Doctor Appointment Log

Provider's Name	Speciality	Reason	Date/Time

MEDICATION TRACKER

Name:

Medication:

Dose & Frequency:

Form:
(Tablet / Syrup / Shot / IV)

Special Instructions:

Date	Time	Reaction

Notes:

Name:

Medication:

Dose & Frequency:

Form:
(Tablet / Syrup / Shot / IV)

Special Instructions:

Date	Time	Reaction

Notes:

Name:

Medication:

Dose & Frequency:

Form:
(Tablet / Syrup / Shot / IV)

Special Instructions:

Date	Time	Reaction

Notes:

MEDICATION TRACKER

Name:	Name:	Name:
Medication:	Medication:	Medication:
Dose & Frequency:	Dose & Frequency:	Dose & Frequency:
Form: (Tablet / Syrup / Shot / IV)	Form: (Tablet / Syrup / Shot / IV)	Form: (Tablet / Syrup / Shot / IV)
Special Instructions:	Special Instructions:	Special Instructions:

Date	Time	Reaction	Date	Time	Reaction	Date	Time	Reaction

Notes:	Notes:	Notes:

MEDICATION TRACKER

Name:

Medication:

Dose & Frequency:

Form:
(Tablet / Syrup / Shot / IV)

Special Instructions:

Date	Time	Reaction

Notes:

Name:

Medication:

Dose & Frequency:

Form:
(Tablet / Syrup / Shot / IV)

Special Instructions:

Date	Time	Reaction

Notes:

Name:

Medication:

Dose & Frequency:

Form:
(Tablet / Syrup / Shot / IV)

Special Instructions:

Date	Time	Reaction

Notes:

MEDICATION TRACKER

Name:	**Name:**	**Name:**
Medication:	**Medication:**	**Medication:**
Dose & Frequency:	**Dose & Frequency:**	**Dose & Frequency:**
Form: (Tablet / Syrup / Shot / IV)	**Form:** (Tablet / Syrup / Shot / IV)	**Form:** (Tablet / Syrup / Shot / IV)
Special Instructions:	**Special Instructions:**	**Special Instructions:**

Date	Time	Reaction	Date	Time	Reaction	Date	Time	Reaction

Notes:	Notes:	Notes:

MEDICATION TRACKER

Name:	Name:	Name:
Medication:	Medication:	Medication:
Dose & Frequency:	Dose & Frequency:	Dose & Frequency:
Form: (Tablet / Syrup / Shot / IV)	Form: (Tablet / Syrup / Shot / IV)	Form: (Tablet / Syrup / Shot / IV)
Special Instructions:	Special Instructions:	Special Instructions:

Date	Time	Reaction	Date	Time	Reaction	Date	Time	Reaction

Notes:	Notes:	Notes:

MEDICATION TRACKER

Name:

Medication:

Dose & Frequency:

Form:
(Tablet / Syrup / Shot / IV)

Special Instructions:

Date	Time	Reaction

Notes:

Name:

Medication:

Dose & Frequency:

Form:
(Tablet / Syrup / Shot / IV)

Special Instructions:

Date	Time	Reaction

Notes:

Name:

Medication:

Dose & Frequency:

Form:
(Tablet / Syrup / Shot / IV)

Special Instructions:

Date	Time	Reaction

Notes:

MEDICATION TRACKER

Name:

Medication:

Dose & Frequency:

Form:
(Tablet / Syrup / Shot / IV)

Special Instructions:

Date	Time	Reaction

Notes:

Name:

Medication:

Dose & Frequency:

Form:
(Tablet / Syrup / Shot / IV)

Special Instructions:

Date	Time	Reaction

Notes:

Name:

Medication:

Dose & Frequency:

Form:
(Tablet / Syrup / Shot / IV)

Special Instructions:

Date	Time	Reaction

Notes:

MEDICATION TRACKER

Name:

Medication:

Dose & Frequency:

Form:
(Tablet / Syrup / Shot / IV)

Special Instructions:

Date	Time	Reaction

Notes:

Name:

Medication:

Dose & Frequency:

Form:
(Tablet / Syrup / Shot / IV)

Special Instructions:

Date	Time	Reaction

Notes:

Name:

Medication:

Dose & Frequency:

Form:
(Tablet / Syrup / Shot / IV)

Special Instructions:

Date	Time	Reaction

Notes:

MEDICATION TRACKER

Name:	Name:	Name:
Medication:	Medication:	Medication:
Dose & Frequency:	Dose & Frequency:	Dose & Frequency:
Form: (Tablet / Syrup / Shot / IV)	Form: (Tablet / Syrup / Shot / IV)	Form: (Tablet / Syrup / Shot / IV)
Special Instructions:	Special Instructions:	Special Instructions:

Date	Time	Reaction	Date	Time	Reaction	Date	Time	Reaction

Notes:	Notes:	Notes:

MEDICATION TRACKER

Name:	Name:	Name:
Medication:	Medication:	Medication:
Dose & Frequency:	Dose & Frequency:	Dose & Frequency:
Form: (Tablet / Syrup / Shot / IV)	Form: (Tablet / Syrup / Shot / IV)	Form: (Tablet / Syrup / Shot / IV)
Special Instructions:	Special Instructions:	Special Instructions:

Date	Time	Reaction	Date	Time	Reaction	Date	Time	Reaction

Notes:	Notes:	Notes:

MEDICATION TRACKER

Name:

Medication:

Dose & Frequency:

Form:
(Tablet / Syrup / Shot / IV)

Special Instructions:

Date	Time	Reaction

Notes:

Name:

Medication:

Dose & Frequency:

Form:
(Tablet / Syrup / Shot / IV)

Special Instructions:

Date	Time	Reaction

Notes:

Name:

Medication:

Dose & Frequency:

Form:
(Tablet / Syrup / Shot / IV)

Special Instructions:

Date	Time	Reaction

Notes:

MEDICATION TRACKER

Name:	Name:	Name:
Medication:	Medication:	Medication:
Dose & Frequency:	Dose & Frequency:	Dose & Frequency:
Form: (Tablet / Syrup / Shot / IV)	Form: (Tablet / Syrup / Shot / IV)	Form: (Tablet / Syrup / Shot / IV)
Special Instructions:	Special Instructions:	Special Instructions:

Date	Time	Reaction	Date	Time	Reaction	Date	Time	Reaction

Notes:	Notes:	Notes:

MEDICATION TRACKER

Name:

Medication:

Dose & Frequency:

Form:
(Tablet / Syrup / Shot / IV)

Special Instructions:

Name:

Medication:

Dose & Frequency:

Form:
(Tablet / Syrup / Shot / IV)

Special Instructions:

Name:

Medication:

Dose & Frequency:

Form:
(Tablet / Syrup / Shot / IV)

Special Instructions:

Date	Time	Reaction	Date	Time	Reaction	Date	Time	Reaction

Notes:

Notes:

Notes:

MEDICATION TRACKER

Name:	Name:	Name:
Medication:	Medication:	Medication:
Dose & Frequency:	Dose & Frequency:	Dose & Frequency:
Form: (Tablet / Syrup / Shot / IV)	Form: (Tablet / Syrup / Shot / IV)	Form: (Tablet / Syrup / Shot / IV)
Special Instructions:	Special Instructions:	Special Instructions:

Date	Time	Reaction	Date	Time	Reaction	Date	Time	Reaction

Notes:	Notes:	Notes:

MEDICATION TRACKER

Name:

Medication:

Dose & Frequency:

Form:
(Tablet / Syrup / Shot / IV)

Special Instructions:

Date	Time	Reaction

Notes:

Name:

Medication:

Dose & Frequency:

Form:
(Tablet / Syrup / Shot / IV)

Special Instructions:

Date	Time	Reaction

Notes:

Name:

Medication:

Dose & Frequency:

Form:
(Tablet / Syrup / Shot / IV)

Special Instructions:

Date	Time	Reaction

Notes:

MEDICATION TRACKER

Name:

Medication:

Dose & Frequency:

Form:
(Tablet / Syrup / Shot / IV)

Special Instructions:

Date	Time	Reaction

Notes:

Name:

Medication:

Dose & Frequency:

Form:
(Tablet / Syrup / Shot / IV)

Special Instructions:

Date	Time	Reaction

Notes:

Name:

Medication:

Dose & Frequency:

Form:
(Tablet / Syrup / Shot / IV)

Special Instructions:

Date	Time	Reaction

Notes:

MEDICATION TRACKER

Name:

Medication:

Dose & Frequency:

Form:
(Tablet / Syrup / Shot / IV)

Special Instructions:

Date	Time	Reaction

Notes:

Name:

Medication:

Dose & Frequency:

Form:
(Tablet / Syrup / Shot / IV)

Special Instructions:

Date	Time	Reaction

Notes:

Name:

Medication:

Dose & Frequency:

Form:
(Tablet / Syrup / Shot / IV)

Special Instructions:

Date	Time	Reaction

Notes:

MEDICATION TRACKER

Name:	Name:	Name:
Medication:	Medication:	Medication:
Dose & Frequency:	Dose & Frequency:	Dose & Frequency:
Form: (Tablet / Syrup / Shot / IV)	Form: (Tablet / Syrup / Shot / IV)	Form: (Tablet / Syrup / Shot / IV)
Special Instructions:	Special Instructions:	Special Instructions:

Date	Time	Reaction	Date	Time	Reaction	Date	Time	Reaction

Notes:	Notes:	Notes:

MEDICATION TRACKER

Name:

Medication:

Dose & Frequency:

Form:
(Tablet / Syrup / Shot / IV)

Special Instructions:

Date	Time	Reaction

Notes:

Name:

Medication:

Dose & Frequency:

Form:
(Tablet / Syrup / Shot / IV)

Special Instructions:

Date	Time	Reaction

Notes:

Name:

Medication:

Dose & Frequency:

Form:
(Tablet / Syrup / Shot / IV)

Special Instructions:

Date	Time	Reaction

Notes:

MEDICATION TRACKER

Name:

Medication:

Dose & Frequency:

Form:
(Tablet / Syrup / Shot / IV)

Special Instructions:

Date	Time	Reaction

Notes:

Name:

Medication:

Dose & Frequency:

Form:
(Tablet / Syrup / Shot / IV)

Special Instructions:

Date	Time	Reaction

Notes:

Name:

Medication:

Dose & Frequency:

Form:
(Tablet / Syrup / Shot / IV)

Special Instructions:

Date	Time	Reaction

Notes:

MEDICATION TRACKER

Name:

Medication:

Dose & Frequency:

Form:
(Tablet / Syrup / Shot / IV)

Special Instructions:

Date	Time	Reaction

Notes:

Name:

Medication:

Dose & Frequency:

Form:
(Tablet / Syrup / Shot / IV)

Special Instructions:

Date	Time	Reaction

Notes:

Name:

Medication:

Dose & Frequency:

Form:
(Tablet / Syrup / Shot / IV)

Special Instructions:

Date	Time	Reaction

Notes:

MEDICATION TRACKER

Name:

Medication:

Dose & Frequency:

Form:
(Tablet / Syrup / Shot / IV)

Special Instructions:

Date	Time	Reaction

Notes:

Name:

Medication:

Dose & Frequency:

Form:
(Tablet / Syrup / Shot / IV)

Special Instructions:

Date	Time	Reaction

Notes:

Name:

Medication:

Dose & Frequency:

Form:
(Tablet / Syrup / Shot / IV)

Special Instructions:

Date	Time	Reaction

Notes:

MEDICATION TRACKER

Name:

Medication:

Dose & Frequency:

Form:
(Tablet / Syrup / Shot / IV)

Special Instructions:

Date	Time	Reaction

Notes:

Name:

Medication:

Dose & Frequency:

Form:
(Tablet / Syrup / Shot / IV)

Special Instructions:

Date	Time	Reaction

Notes:

Name:

Medication:

Dose & Frequency:

Form:
(Tablet / Syrup / Shot / IV)

Special Instructions:

Date	Time	Reaction

Notes:

MEDICATION TRACKER

Name:

Medication:

Dose & Frequency:

Form:
(Tablet / Syrup / Shot / IV)

Special Instructions:

Date	Time	Reaction

Notes:

Name:

Medication:

Dose & Frequency:

Form:
(Tablet / Syrup / Shot / IV)

Special Instructions:

Date	Time	Reaction

Notes:

Name:

Medication:

Dose & Frequency:

Form:
(Tablet / Syrup / Shot / IV)

Special Instructions:

Date	Time	Reaction

Notes:

MEDICATION TRACKER

Name:

Medication:

Dose & Frequency:

Form:
(Tablet / Syrup / Shot / IV)

Special Instructions:

Date	Time	Reaction

Notes:

Name:

Medication:

Dose & Frequency:

Form:
(Tablet / Syrup / Shot / IV)

Special Instructions:

Date	Time	Reaction

Notes:

Name:

Medication:

Dose & Frequency:

Form:
(Tablet / Syrup / Shot / IV)

Special Instructions:

Date	Time	Reaction

Notes:

MEDICATION TRACKER

Name:

Medication:

Dose & Frequency:

Form:
(Tablet / Syrup / Shot / IV)

Special Instructions:

Date	Time	Reaction

Notes:

Name:

Medication:

Dose & Frequency:

Form:
(Tablet / Syrup / Shot / IV)

Special Instructions:

Date	Time	Reaction

Notes:

Name:

Medication:

Dose & Frequency:

Form:
(Tablet / Syrup / Shot / IV)

Special Instructions:

Date	Time	Reaction

Notes:

MEDICATION TRACKER

Name:

Medication:

Dose & Frequency:

Form:
(Tablet / Syrup / Shot / IV)

Special Instructions:

Date	Time	Reaction

Notes:

Name:

Medication:

Dose & Frequency:

Form:
(Tablet / Syrup / Shot / IV)

Special Instructions:

Date	Time	Reaction

Notes:

Name:

Medication:

Dose & Frequency:

Form:
(Tablet / Syrup / Shot / IV)

Special Instructions:

Date	Time	Reaction

Notes:

MEDICATION TRACKER

Name:

Medication:

Dose & Frequency:

Form:
(Tablet / Syrup / Shot / IV)

Special Instructions:

Date	Time	Reaction

Notes:

Name:

Medication:

Dose & Frequency:

Form:
(Tablet / Syrup / Shot / IV)

Special Instructions:

Date	Time	Reaction

Notes:

Name:

Medication:

Dose & Frequency:

Form:
(Tablet / Syrup / Shot / IV)

Special Instructions:

Date	Time	Reaction

Notes:

MEDICATION TRACKER

Name:

Medication:

Dose & Frequency:

Form:
(Tablet / Syrup / Shot / IV)

Special Instructions:

Name:

Medication:

Dose & Frequency:

Form:
(Tablet / Syrup / Shot / IV)

Special Instructions:

Name:

Medication:

Dose & Frequency:

Form:
(Tablet / Syrup / Shot / IV)

Special Instructions:

Date	Time	Reaction	Date	Time	Reaction	Date	Time	Reaction

Notes:

Notes:

Notes:

MEDICATION TRACKER

Name:	Name:	Name:
Medication:	Medication:	Medication:
Dose & Frequency:	Dose & Frequency:	Dose & Frequency:
Form: (Tablet / Syrup / Shot / IV)	Form: (Tablet / Syrup / Shot / IV)	Form: (Tablet / Syrup / Shot / IV)
Special Instructions:	Special Instructions:	Special Instructions:

Date	Time	Reaction	Date	Time	Reaction	Date	Time	Reaction

Notes:	Notes:	Notes:

MEDICATION TRACKER

Name:

Medication:

Dose & Frequency:

Form:
(Tablet / Syrup / Shot / IV)

Special Instructions:

Date	Time	Reaction

Notes:

Name:

Medication:

Dose & Frequency:

Form:
(Tablet / Syrup / Shot / IV)

Special Instructions:

Date	Time	Reaction

Notes:

Name:

Medication:

Dose & Frequency:

Form:
(Tablet / Syrup / Shot / IV)

Special Instructions:

Date	Time	Reaction

Notes:

MEDICATION TRACKER

Name:	Name:	Name:
Medication:	Medication:	Medication:
Dose & Frequency:	Dose & Frequency:	Dose & Frequency:
Form: (Tablet / Syrup / Shot / IV)	Form: (Tablet / Syrup / Shot / IV)	Form: (Tablet / Syrup / Shot / IV)
Special Instructions:	Special Instructions:	Special Instructions:

Date	Time	Reaction	Date	Time	Reaction	Date	Time	Reaction

Notes:	Notes:	Notes:

MEDICATION TRACKER

Name:

Medication:

Dose & Frequency:

Form:
(Tablet / Syrup / Shot / IV)

Special Instructions:

Date	Time	Reaction

Notes:

Name:

Medication:

Dose & Frequency:

Form:
(Tablet / Syrup / Shot / IV)

Special Instructions:

Date	Time	Reaction

Notes:

Name:

Medication:

Dose & Frequency:

Form:
(Tablet / Syrup / Shot / IV)

Special Instructions:

Date	Time	Reaction

Notes:

MEDICATION TRACKER

Name:	Name:	Name:
Medication:	Medication:	Medication:
Dose & Frequency:	Dose & Frequency:	Dose & Frequency:
Form: (Tablet / Syrup / Shot / IV)	Form: (Tablet / Syrup / Shot / IV)	Form: (Tablet / Syrup / Shot / IV)
Special Instructions:	Special Instructions:	Special Instructions:

Date	Time	Reaction	Date	Time	Reaction	Date	Time	Reaction

Notes:	Notes:	Notes:

MEDICATION TRACKER

Name:

Medication:

Dose & Frequency:

Form:
(Tablet / Syrup / Shot / IV)

Special Instructions:

Date	Time	Reaction

Notes:

Name:

Medication:

Dose & Frequency:

Form:
(Tablet / Syrup / Shot / IV)

Special Instructions:

Date	Time	Reaction

Notes:

Name:

Medication:

Dose & Frequency:

Form:
(Tablet / Syrup / Shot / IV)

Special Instructions:

Date	Time	Reaction

Notes:

MEDICATION TRACKER

Name:	Name:	Name:
Medication:	Medication:	Medication:
Dose & Frequency:	Dose & Frequency:	Dose & Frequency:
Form: (Tablet / Syrup / Shot / IV)	Form: (Tablet / Syrup / Shot / IV)	Form: (Tablet / Syrup / Shot / IV)
Special Instructions:	Special Instructions:	Special Instructions:

Date	Time	Reaction	Date	Time	Reaction	Date	Time	Reaction

Notes:	Notes:	Notes:

MEDICATION TRACKER

Name:

Medication:

Dose & Frequency:

Form:
(Tablet / Syrup / Shot / IV)

Special Instructions:

Name:

Medication:

Dose & Frequency:

Form:
(Tablet / Syrup / Shot / IV)

Special Instructions:

Name:

Medication:

Dose & Frequency:

Form:
(Tablet / Syrup / Shot / IV)

Special Instructions:

Date	Time	Reaction	Date	Time	Reaction	Date	Time	Reaction

Notes:

Notes:

Notes:

MEDICATION TRACKER

Name:

Medication:

Dose & Frequency:

Form:
(Tablet / Syrup / Shot / IV)

Special Instructions:

Date	Time	Reaction

Notes:

Name:

Medication:

Dose & Frequency:

Form:
(Tablet / Syrup / Shot / IV)

Special Instructions:

Date	Time	Reaction

Notes:

Name:

Medication:

Dose & Frequency:

Form:
(Tablet / Syrup / Shot / IV)

Special Instructions:

Date	Time	Reaction

Notes:

MEDICATION TRACKER

Name:

Medication:

Dose & Frequency:

Form:
(Tablet / Syrup / Shot / IV)

Special Instructions:

Date	Time	Reaction

Notes:

Name:

Medication:

Dose & Frequency:

Form:
(Tablet / Syrup / Shot / IV)

Special Instructions:

Date	Time	Reaction

Notes:

Name:

Medication:

Dose & Frequency:

Form:
(Tablet / Syrup / Shot / IV)

Special Instructions:

Date	Time	Reaction

Notes:

MEDICATION TRACKER

Name:	Name:	Name:
Medication:	Medication:	Medication:
Dose & Frequency:	Dose & Frequency:	Dose & Frequency:
Form: (Tablet / Syrup / Shot / IV)	Form: (Tablet / Syrup / Shot / IV)	Form: (Tablet / Syrup / Shot / IV)
Special Instructions:	Special Instructions:	Special Instructions:

Date	Time	Reaction	Date	Time	Reaction	Date	Time	Reaction

Notes:	Notes:	Notes:

MEDICATION TRACKER

Name:

Medication:

Dose & Frequency:

Form:
(Tablet / Syrup / Shot / IV)

Special Instructions:

Date	Time	Reaction

Notes:

Name:

Medication:

Dose & Frequency:

Form:
(Tablet / Syrup / Shot / IV)

Special Instructions:

Date	Time	Reaction

Notes:

Name:

Medication:

Dose & Frequency:

Form:
(Tablet / Syrup / Shot / IV)

Special Instructions:

Date	Time	Reaction

Notes:

MEDICATION TRACKER

Name:

Medication:

Dose & Frequency:

Form:
(Tablet / Syrup / Shot / IV)

Special Instructions:

Name:

Medication:

Dose & Frequency:

Form:
(Tablet / Syrup / Shot / IV)

Special Instructions:

Name:

Medication:

Dose & Frequency:

Form:
(Tablet / Syrup / Shot / IV)

Special Instructions:

Date	Time	Reaction	Date	Time	Reaction	Date	Time	Reaction

Notes:	Notes:	Notes:

MEDICATION TRACKER

Name:

Medication:

Dose & Frequency:

Form:
(Tablet / Syrup / Shot / IV)

Special Instructions:

Date	Time	Reaction

Notes:

Name:

Medication:

Dose & Frequency:

Form:
(Tablet / Syrup / Shot / IV)

Special Instructions:

Date	Time	Reaction

Notes:

Name:

Medication:

Dose & Frequency:

Form:
(Tablet / Syrup / Shot / IV)

Special Instructions:

Date	Time	Reaction

Notes:

MEDICATION TRACKER

Name:

Medication:

Dose & Frequency:

Form:
(Tablet / Syrup / Shot / IV)

Special Instructions:

Date	Time	Reaction

Notes:

Name:

Medication:

Dose & Frequency:

Form:
(Tablet / Syrup / Shot / IV)

Special Instructions:

Date	Time	Reaction

Notes:

Name:

Medication:

Dose & Frequency:

Form:
(Tablet / Syrup / Shot / IV)

Special Instructions:

Date	Time	Reaction

Notes:

MEDICATION TRACKER

Name:	**Name:**	**Name:**
Medication:	**Medication:**	**Medication:**
Dose & Frequency:	**Dose & Frequency:**	**Dose & Frequency:**
Form: (Tablet / Syrup / Shot / IV)	**Form:** (Tablet / Syrup / Shot / IV)	**Form:** (Tablet / Syrup / Shot / IV)
Special Instructions:	**Special Instructions:**	**Special Instructions:**

Date	Time	Reaction	Date	Time	Reaction	Date	Time	Reaction

Notes:	**Notes:**	**Notes:**

MEDICATION TRACKER

Name:	Name:	Name:
Medication:	Medication:	Medication:
Dose & Frequency:	Dose & Frequency:	Dose & Frequency:
Form: (Tablet / Syrup / Shot / IV)	Form: (Tablet / Syrup / Shot / IV)	Form: (Tablet / Syrup / Shot / IV)
Special Instructions:	Special Instructions:	Special Instructions:

Date	Time	Reaction	Date	Time	Reaction	Date	Time	Reaction

Notes:	Notes:	Notes:

MEDICATION TRACKER

Name:

Medication:

Dose & Frequency:

Form:
(Tablet / Syrup / Shot / IV)

Special Instructions:

Date	Time	Reaction

Notes:

Name:

Medication:

Dose & Frequency:

Form:
(Tablet / Syrup / Shot / IV)

Special Instructions:

Date	Time	Reaction

Notes:

Name:

Medication:

Dose & Frequency:

Form:
(Tablet / Syrup / Shot / IV)

Special Instructions:

Date	Time	Reaction

Notes:

MEDICATION TRACKER

Name:	Name:	Name:
Medication:	Medication:	Medication:
Dose & Frequency:	Dose & Frequency:	Dose & Frequency:
Form: (Tablet / Syrup / Shot / IV)	Form: (Tablet / Syrup / Shot / IV)	Form: (Tablet / Syrup / Shot / IV)
Special Instructions:	Special Instructions:	Special Instructions:

Date	Time	Reaction	Date	Time	Reaction	Date	Time	Reaction

Notes:	Notes:	Notes:

MEDICATION TRACKER

Name:

Medication:

Dose & Frequency:

Form:
(Tablet / Syrup / Shot / IV)

Special Instructions:

Date	Time	Reaction

Notes:

Name:

Medication:

Dose & Frequency:

Form:
(Tablet / Syrup / Shot / IV)

Special Instructions:

Date	Time	Reaction

Notes:

Name:

Medication:

Dose & Frequency:

Form:
(Tablet / Syrup / Shot / IV)

Special Instructions:

Date	Time	Reaction

Notes:

MEDICATION TRACKER

Name:	Name:	Name:
Medication:	Medication:	Medication:
Dose & Frequency:	Dose & Frequency:	Dose & Frequency:
Form: (Tablet / Syrup / Shot / IV)	Form: (Tablet / Syrup / Shot / IV)	Form: (Tablet / Syrup / Shot / IV)
Special Instructions:	Special Instructions:	Special Instructions:

Date	Time	Reaction	Date	Time	Reaction	Date	Time	Reaction

Notes:	Notes:	Notes:

MEDICATION TRACKER

Name:	Name:	Name:
Medication:	Medication:	Medication:
Dose & Frequency:	Dose & Frequency:	Dose & Frequency:
Form: (Tablet / Syrup / Shot / IV)	Form: (Tablet / Syrup / Shot / IV)	Form: (Tablet / Syrup / Shot / IV)
Special Instructions:	Special Instructions:	Special Instructions:

Date	Time	Reaction	Date	Time	Reaction	Date	Time	Reaction

Notes:	Notes:	Notes:

MEDICATION TRACKER

Name:	Name:	Name:
Medication:	Medication:	Medication:
Dose & Frequency:	Dose & Frequency:	Dose & Frequency:
Form: (Tablet / Syrup / Shot / IV)	Form: (Tablet / Syrup / Shot / IV)	Form: (Tablet / Syrup / Shot / IV)
Special Instructions:	Special Instructions:	Special Instructions:

Date	Time	Reaction	Date	Time	Reaction	Date	Time	Reaction

Notes:	Notes:	Notes:

MEDICATION TRACKER

Name:

Medication:

Dose & Frequency:

Form:
(Tablet / Syrup / Shot / IV)

Special Instructions:

Date	Time	Reaction

Notes:

Name:

Medication:

Dose & Frequency:

Form:
(Tablet / Syrup / Shot / IV)

Special Instructions:

Date	Time	Reaction

Notes:

Name:

Medication:

Dose & Frequency:

Form:
(Tablet / Syrup / Shot / IV)

Special Instructions:

Date	Time	Reaction

Notes:

MEDICATION TRACKER

Name:	Name:	Name:
Medication:	Medication:	Medication:
Dose & Frequency:	Dose & Frequency:	Dose & Frequency:
Form: (Tablet / Syrup / Shot / IV)	Form: (Tablet / Syrup / Shot / IV)	Form: (Tablet / Syrup / Shot / IV)
Special Instructions:	Special Instructions:	Special Instructions:

Date	Time	Reaction	Date	Time	Reaction	Date	Time	Reaction

Notes:	Notes:	Notes:

MEDICATION TRACKER

Name:

Medication:

Dose & Frequency:

Form:
(Tablet / Syrup / Shot / IV)

Special Instructions:

Name:

Medication:

Dose & Frequency:

Form:
(Tablet / Syrup / Shot / IV)

Special Instructions:

Name:

Medication:

Dose & Frequency:

Form:
(Tablet / Syrup / Shot / IV)

Special Instructions:

Date	Time	Reaction	Date	Time	Reaction	Date	Time	Reaction

Notes:

Notes:

Notes:

MEDICATION TRACKER

Name:

Medication:

Dose & Frequency:

Form:
(Tablet / Syrup / Shot / IV)

Special Instructions:

Date	Time	Reaction

Notes:

Name:

Medication:

Dose & Frequency:

Form:
(Tablet / Syrup / Shot / IV)

Special Instructions:

Date	Time	Reaction

Notes:

Name:

Medication:

Dose & Frequency:

Form:
(Tablet / Syrup / Shot / IV)

Special Instructions:

Date	Time	Reaction

Notes:

MEDICATION TRACKER

Name:

Medication:

Dose & Frequency:

Form:
(Tablet / Syrup / Shot / IV)

Special Instructions:

Date	Time	Reaction

Notes:

Name:

Medication:

Dose & Frequency:

Form:
(Tablet / Syrup / Shot / IV)

Special Instructions:

Date	Time	Reaction

Notes:

Name:

Medication:

Dose & Frequency:

Form:
(Tablet / Syrup / Shot / IV)

Special Instructions:

Date	Time	Reaction

Notes:

MEDICATION TRACKER

Name:	Name:	Name:
Medication:	Medication:	Medication:
Dose & Frequency:	Dose & Frequency:	Dose & Frequency:
Form: (Tablet / Syrup / Shot / IV)	Form: (Tablet / Syrup / Shot / IV)	Form: (Tablet / Syrup / Shot / IV)
Special Instructions:	Special Instructions:	Special Instructions:

Date	Time	Reaction	Date	Time	Reaction	Date	Time	Reaction

Notes:	Notes:	Notes:

MEDICATION TRACKER

Name:	Name:	Name:
Medication:	Medication:	Medication:
Dose & Frequency:	Dose & Frequency:	Dose & Frequency:
Form: (Tablet / Syrup / Shot / IV)	Form: (Tablet / Syrup / Shot / IV)	Form: (Tablet / Syrup / Shot / IV)
Special Instructions:	Special Instructions:	Special Instructions:

Date	Time	Reaction	Date	Time	Reaction	Date	Time	Reaction

Notes:	Notes:	Notes:

MEDICATION TRACKER

Name:

Medication:

Dose & Frequency:

Form:
(Tablet / Syrup / Shot / IV)

Special Instructions:

Date	Time	Reaction

Notes:

Name:

Medication:

Dose & Frequency:

Form:
(Tablet / Syrup / Shot / IV)

Special Instructions:

Date	Time	Reaction

Notes:

Name:

Medication:

Dose & Frequency:

Form:
(Tablet / Syrup / Shot / IV)

Special Instructions:

Date	Time	Reaction

Notes:

MEDICATION TRACKER

Name:

Medication:

Dose & Frequency:

Form:
(Tablet / Syrup / Shot / IV)

Special Instructions:

Date	Time	Reaction

Notes:

Name:

Medication:

Dose & Frequency:

Form:
(Tablet / Syrup / Shot / IV)

Special Instructions:

Date	Time	Reaction

Notes:

Name:

Medication:

Dose & Frequency:

Form:
(Tablet / Syrup / Shot / IV)

Special Instructions:

Date	Time	Reaction

Notes:

NOTES

Name:

NOTES

Name:

NOTES

Name:

NOTES

Name:

NOTES

Name:

NOTES

Name:

NOTES

Name:

NOTES

Name:

STAY ORGANIZED
STAY EMPOWERED

Want a FREE Healthy Meal Planner?

Get your free printable, plus health tips to help you stay on track.

Visit: www.mealplan.adalynnjames.com
Enter your name & email to download instantly!

Enjoying this logbook?

Your honest review helps others find this book and supports businesses like ours.

Please take a minute to leave a review on Amazon.
We read every single one! Scan the QR code below.

https://bit.ly/FamilyMedsBookReview

— DigiMedical, by Adalynn James Publishing

Digi Medical

ADALYNN JAMES

Made in United States
Cleveland, OH
04 November 2026

47647246R00045